THE TRUTH ABOUT WITCHES

# THE TRUTH
## ABOUT WITCHES

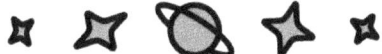

DIFFERENTIATING FACT
FROM SOCIETAL NORMS

Marianne Maciborski

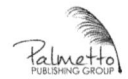

Palmetto Publishing Group
Charleston, SC

*The Truth About Witches*
Copyright © 2020 by Marianne Maciborski
All rights reserved

No portion of this book may be reproduced, stored in a retrieval system, or transmitted in any form by any means–electronic, mechanical, photocopy, recording, or other except for brief quotations in printed reviews, without prior permission of the author.

First Edition

Printed in the United States

ISBN-13: 978-1-64111-706-7
ISBN-10: 1-64111-706-0

*For confidentiality purposes, some names have been changed.*

*Disclaimer: I blame no one for nothing, but instead the amount of misinformation out there.*

*This book is dedicated to Margaret "Maggie" McCullough and Rita Hays, thank you for teaching me more than I ever knew about myself.*

# CHAPTER ONE

I KNEW IT FROM THE DAY I TURNED EIGH-teen. I knew that somehow I was different. Prior to now I just never put two and two together and in the years following I would come to find that I knew so much more.

Prior to starting college in late August 2001, I fell subject to years of conformity and silence. I had very little say in my life, and if I was allowed to make a choice or provide input it was often about frivolous matters. My silence, as I now realize, was mainly due to the fact that I am an indigo adult as well as a modern-day witch. Still, when I started college I was allowed to come alive, for a few brief years; before being somewhat silenced again, but this is when the realization came. I realized that events that happened in my life up until now were not just happenstance and to some extent, Universe would have rather had me dead but for reasons, good and bad, coexisting in time-space allowed me to stay alive to complete my mission of both learning and teaching on this planet.

Sometime in the late 90s I indirectly learned that allopathic medicine helped me to recover as best I could, or so they said, and Universe now just left me to "run amuck" and make what I could out of my life, however still not wanting anything to do with my life I casually pushed that thought aside and just figured I would see how far I could run before something truly did happen. Up until now I had been artificially propelled through life and while I was allowed to "come alive" these last few years and develop a sense of self it seemed as though people in some authoritative position in my life were telling me what to do. I had two degrees still I was not sure that I wanted to utilize either one of them, at least not the way that college intended, and instead wanted to pursue my interest in alternative media to see where that took me.

"Look for a job," and "work more" are two of the key phrases that I heard continually echoed by my parents and still I wanted neither of these as up until now I was forced to conform and while college did give me some room to be me I was still forced to conform in some way. A job in the corporate sector meant conformity in some way; and working more in my job, or any other job for that matter, meant agreeing to be treated like a number or a disposable at best. With this said I quickly learned how to lead two lives, one in which I looked at alternative material and the other where I dealt with the harshness of reality. Still my thoughts and answers were now primarily based on how I saw things from an alternative standpoint so my views were very rarely those of the corporate sector. Thus said job interviews created an awkward feeling for me as prior to going in I already knew I was not going to get the job based on my differing views. Still by this time I put up a façade just to keep the job I had. While I continued job hunting the overall hunt grew less and less as I went further into exploring alternative media and began seeing just how corrupt some parts of the corporate sector really were. Finally in early 2012 I stopped job hunting all together after one job interview left me totally speechless. My initial words to the four-walled room where I was sitting were "corporate America can go sit and spin on it, and I will deal with them when I am ready to deal with them." After that, I stared blankly at my computer screen. I had two degrees which at this point I considered useless and already felt like a failure in life so what was I going to do now? Thoughts ran wild in my head for a few brief moments and then my mind came to rest on the thought that I developed in 2008 when I put my Bioness unit on my leg for the first time, "and this too is only temporary." I paused and then repeated these words over and over in my mind. While I experienced setbacks before this too was only a setback and nothing that I could not overcome. Would it take longer than things in the past? Most definitely yes, still it was something that I could overcome. By this time I knew enough about the alternative sector to know that there were alternative means for healing and I just had to seek them out. After all the way I figured it if Universe could keep the reality of what is going on a secret then why not keep the truth about your own health a secret too? I stumbled upon one name and then another, and by this time I began figuring if Universe did not want me the way I was then I would just focus on taking care of myself and guess what, sooner or later a whole new world would open up. Eventually, I managed to get in touch with a Naturopath who started me out on his program and after doing several cleanses things started coming out of my body. Still having a strong connection to the allopathic medical model I quickly contacted my Naturopath and eventually set up a time and place to meet. My Mother not wanting to know the truth did not go but my Dad, seeing that I was trying to better myself, agreed to take me even though the appointment involved travel.

While I was still skeptic into the Naturopathic work that this doctor did as the whole thing did entail a fairly large sum of money I resolved prior to and after making the appointment I would go and if I gained something from the whole meeting it was worth it; if I found that it was just a bunch of hooey nonsense then I only wasted my time and money once, after all I had taken two prescription drugs earlier in the year that almost killed me so what is the worst that could happen? Finally, the day came for my appointment and Dad and I left the house mid-morning as my appointment was not till 1 pm and we were going back an hour with the time zone change. By this time I have to say that I felt just a little bit excited as I looked at this doctors' work enough online to feel like I was not going to be disappointed. When we arrived in St. Louis where my appointment was we had about an hour before I had to be there. This gave us time to figure out exactly where we were going and then relax in the lobby of the hotel where my appointment was. We did not eat lunch as I could not eat an hour before my appointment and honestly I have to say that I was not hungry anyway. By now I was too excited knowing that I was doing the right thing and more so knowing that I was going to change my life forever. A few more minutes passed and then my Naturopathic doctor walked into the lobby to take me upstairs. He walked over and introduced himself as Gary Tunsky and said that he was the Naturopath that I had spoken to and set up an appointment with. From there my Dad and I followed him upstairs to where his hotel room was. Now I was starting to get a little nervous as I realized if this whole thing really was a bunch of hooey I would get to look like a fool in front of my Dad and not only would I feel bad but he would feel bad for me. As we walked I quickly pushed that thought out of my mind and began wondering what the whole scan would entail. While I watched multiple videos online from Gary (one directly talking about the scan he used), seeing a video was one thing and seeing it done in person was another. Once we made it to Gary's room and we were all inside I saw his wife, Renee, getting things back together after their last patient. Gary first talked to me for a few minutes and my Dad filled in some blanks of things that I could not remember since my brain aneurysm, then things started. First Gary did his portion of the scan where he was able to see what was going on inside of my body and make suggestions as to things that I could do to help improve them. Next was the Biofeedback portion of the appointment. Once this scan was complete and the report was printed Gary went over the report with me while Renee went out to run some errands. Initially Renee seemed in a little of a hurry to leave, and while I quickly picked up on this and why, I was not alarmed. I had done enough research prior to now to figure out that I was vaccine injured still now was not the time to bring that question into the light as there were more pressing issues that needed to be addressed.

# CHAPTER TWO

AFTER RENEE LEFT GARY SAT DOWN TO GO over the scan report with me and the whole thing, unlike any medical exam, took about two hours. Looking back now it is funny to think how a Naturopath can spend forty-five minutes to an hour gathering information and then two hours going over it while any kind of medical doctor will walk in the room and you will be lucky if they are in the room for five minutes. Walking back down to the lobby with Gary I have to say that I did feel a lot better about life knowing that I did not have to continue giving myself up to the medical paradigm and that I could, in fact, control my own health. Once we made it back down to the lobby Gary told us goodbye and we left. Dad and I got into the van to head home and after we had been driving for ten or fifteen minutes in silence my Dad made a comment about what Gary said about why I had my aneurysm. The comment shocked me and I almost said something back but then I remembered we still had the remainder of the three-hour drive so to keep the peace I just kept my mouth shut. What Gary said made a whole lot more sense than the doctor's explanation that I was just one in a really big number; and for that matter, I thought, will we ever really know the whole truth? My Dad made the comment that I had a lot of things to think about but at least I had a place to start. Gary suggested that I look into getting my Atlas adjusted after my scan and since I knew from previous research that the Atlas affects balance I knew that was where I was going to start. Having been given the NUCCA website I figured I would look at that tomorrow and hope there was a chiropractor in the area and send an email then after I had that whole process going I would worry about everything else.

The next morning I woke at my usual time, dressed and did my usual routine. Once both of my parents left and I finished taking care of things around the house I sat down to look at the NUCCA website. I found that there were no NUCCA chiropractors within a reasonable distance from where I lived, however, the website did bring up three. They were all a three-hour drive, but I figured on a long shot if Dad knew that it would help me he may agree to take me. There were two chiropractors in Indiana and the third was in Paducah, Kentucky. I went ahead and sent emails to all three of them and just figured I would talk to Dad when he came home that afternoon since I wanted to get things started as quickly as possible. When Dad came home I explained that there were three chiropractors in our area that adjusted the Atlas. Two of them were in Indiana and the other in Paducah, Kentucky. The ones in Indiana were in Noblesville and Warsaw. Paducah, which was closer, did involve the hour time change, but that is the one I would probably choose. Still having already emailed all three it was a wait and see to see which chiropractor I would hear back from first before I would make my next move. That evening I checked my email just to see if there was any "good news." It turned out all three chiropractors answered me back. The chiropractor in Noblesville said yes I should have my Atlas adjusted, the chiropractor in Warsaw had a corrupted website and the chiropractor in Paducah sensing I was not from the area asked where I lived and he would try to help me locate a chiropractor closer to me that did the same thing. I called Dad and let him read David's response. After reading it Dad told me to let him know where I lived but if there was not a chiropractor closer that I would come to see him. After sending him my response I shut down my computer and went to bed. I felt like I accomplished something, and while it ultimately may mean more travel if that is what it had to be then that is what it had to be. My life had been like this too long and thankfully my Dad could see that the medical system was not giving me answers but instead just trying to shove more medicine in me that really was not going to heal me anyway.

The next morning after my parents were gone I checked my email and saw that David already responded to me. I opened the email with great anticipation figuring either there was something closer to me or we would be making the three-hour trek down to Paducah at least two or three times. It turned out that there was an Atlas Orthongist less than fifteen minutes away from me the only difference was instead of using hands to fix the problem they used a machine. This place David said was called Louisville Spinal Care and he recommended Dr. Sammi Segal. After reading this I looked up Louisville Spinal Care online and sent them an email. Feeling satisfied I now had a working answer for my Atlas I began looking at the other things that Gary and I talked about. I quickly made the decision that the pieces of equipment Gary suggested that I purchase from him were just going to be temporary fixes and something that I would continually have to do day after day to maintain anything. What I decided I needed to focus on was the supplements or the cell restoration products that Gary recommended, plus the restoration products were much cheaper too. I started looking at every product online by typing the name in to see what links came up I would often end up looking at multiple websites that came up but by doing this for all of Gary's recommendations I quickly narrowed down what I wanted to focus on improving in my body and in the coming days I placed my order with his shipping department. After I placed my first order I realized that the restoration products were not all that cheap either, but I figured if they worked I would keep using them. The way I figured it the scan proved to give solid results so I figured I probably would not be disappointed with the products either.

Two days passed and I received a call back from Louisville Spinal Care, not an email but a phone call. Without hesitation, I went ahead and set up my consultation as Dad and I already talked about a time and once my appointment was made all that was left to do was sit back and wait. My consultation was scheduled for August 19, 2015, about five weeks after I saw Gary. While I was skeptical going into the appointment I knew that my life was going to change for the better one way or another. The consult took about thirty minutes and the x-rays took somewhere between fifteen and twenty minutes then my Dad and I were free to leave since my appointment to come in and go over the x-rays and start treatment was already made. I came in on Friday to go over the x-rays and get my first treatment and then Dr. Segal said that they would put some Kinesio tape on my back as that was something they were experimenting with for their patients and then he said wanted me to come in for two adjustments the following week. Once I was done with Dr. Segal I waited for my taping. I did schedule my two appointments for the following week while I waited and then I thought about this whole idea of Kinesio tape. While I knew what the tape was for I thought "why did I agree to this? I know it is not going to help and in the end just be a waste of my time." When I did finally see the worker who was doing the taping he looked like some kid right out of college who did not have too much of a clue what he was doing as he had to keep looking in a book throughout the whole process and when the whole thing was done it actually took longer than the appointment. I wore the Kinesio tape till my first appointment the following week and long story short it did absolutely nothing accept cause a whole lot of discomfort. The tape was taken off at my next appointment and I did not need my Atlas adjusted so the Kinesio tape was just put on again, following a different diagram, and all the while I was thinking "what if it was that easy, what if I was adjusted once and now my Atlas is going to hold." I quickly snapped out of that thought though as the whole taping process started, and right away I thought "I know I am going to gain nothing again but at least this is the last time I will be taped." The whole taping ordeal as Dr. Segal explained was only something they did twice and for my sake thankfully that was it as I gained nothing and felt like it was a big waste of time. Going back in that week the tape was removed and I wound up not needing to be adjusted that day either. I made my appointments for the following week and then my Dad and I left. I thought little more about the chiropractor that day and when I really did start to think about things the following day my first thought was "how can it be that easy?" My Atlas had been out of alignment since 1987, there is no way that after just one adjustment my Atlas was going to be fixed. Still looking back now I have to wonder if that was some part of the attempt to give me false hope.

# CHAPTER THREE

SOON ENOUGH THE FOLLOWING WEEK MY first appointment came. I knew that Dr. Segal, or Sammi as I now called him in my mind, was going to adjust me based on the pop I felt in my neck on Sunday while I was at work. Sammi walked in the room and the first thing I said was "you are going to adjust me." The conversation went on and yes Sammi did wind up adjusting my Atlas and after that held he adjusted the rest of my back with the impulse gun. My following appointment Sammi adjusted my Atlas twice, and that is when looking back I have to say it all began. Sammi would adjust my Atlas for so many appointments then not adjust it, he would use the impulse gun sometimes and not others, and sometimes he would do neither. I did not think much of this erratic pattern at first I was just glad when Sammi said I could start coming once a week as quickly as he did. While Sammi's job was to adjust my Atlas we did have multiple other conversations and at some point early on in my treatment, probably during the fourth week, Sammi made mention of the fact that over adjustment can cause nerve damage. Looking back if I could go back to that day I would have walked out of the room right then and changed chiropractors, but I did not somehow thinking that Sammi's erratic patterns would change and subliminally sensing Sammi needed something like this right then.

The erratic patterns in my treatment continued, however as time progressed grew to having my Atlas adjusted multiple times. There were times I had my Atlas adjusted two, three and even four times and many of these appointments, other than my first few appointments I had no pain in my neck. There were times, I remember, when Sammi would stand there palpating my neck for five or more minutes just to find some reason to adjust my Atlas when nothing hurt at all. This is when I really began to communicate with Gary. Not that I ever stopped communicating with him since my appointment in July but this is really when I began asking questions. Sammi noted early on in my treatment that he looked only at the Atlas thus I learned early on that when I asked a question, not related to the Atlas, his favorite phrase was "I don't know." Never once did I hear "I will look into that," and I quickly learned just to do the research myself ahead of time or talk things through with Gary beforehand. I would often just ask

Sammi questions to create an awkward feeling and later on, it became just for kicks.

Feeling frustrated with not knowing why Sammi continually adjusted me even when I felt like I did not need it I finally emailed Gary in late August to find out if there was something else my body needed other than to have my Atlas adjusted. I figured whatever Gary's answer was it did not mean I would stop going to the chiropractor I just would simply add it to the mix. As crazy as my life was at this point, thanks to Sammi, what difference would a new treatment make? When Gary replied he said that I needed cranial sacral therapy too. "That is easy enough," I thought and enthusiastically began research into the therapy. Once I found out the basics of what this therapy did I quickly saw that these therapists could treat more than just TMJ as I now had other areas of pain in my body too. Still, when I began looking for a Craniosacral therapist I found that many of them practice out of their house, and when I did find therapists that practiced out of some sort of office I was overjoyed. I immediately told my Dad what Gary said and as in the past, he told me just to go ahead and make an appointment. Long story short I decided to wait and talk things over with Sammi first and what a mistake that was. When I told Sammi what Gary said he just about flew out of his skin and almost threw his iPad. After a few moments, I guess he composed himself enough to raise his voice, what little he could, and pointing at the orthogonal machine by which I was sitting said, "if I can adjust you with this, then that is all you need." I said okay, flipped myself around on the table and walked out.

When I made it to the front my Dad proceeded to pay, I made my next appointment and we walked out. After we were out of the building my Dad asked 'so what did Sammi say about Craniosacral therapy?"

"I do not need it," I replied.

After that, my Dad did not say anything else the rest of the way home. Thankfully, as this gave me time to think; if Sammi became that defensive about me trying a different modality of treatment what was he trying to hide? When we arrived home I resolved not to think about this anymore until the following day. Morning came and soon enough my parents left for work. Once I finished doing things around the house and I sat down to do things for me. I emailed the three Craniosacral therapists I found on the Internet that were within a reasonable distance from where I lived. The first therapist to answer back also listed some times in the next two weeks that she had available. Right then I was sold and the best part was she was only a short distance from the house. I sent an email back and wound up taking a 4 pm appointment the following week. At this point, I had not heard back from the other two Craniosacral therapists and figured if I did I just would not pursue them any further. Later that day I received another email from my Craniosacral therapist with my paperwork attached which I printed and filled out that way I would have that much longer for my appointment.

When my appointment came the following week I asked my Dad if he would take me as I did not know exactly what it would entail. When we arrived and opened the office door I noticed that the waiting room was very different as there was no receptionist and the waiting area itself was much smaller than most offices I had been in. Soon enough though my therapist appeared and introduced herself as Gina Flowers. Gina was a middle-aged woman with a pleasant demeanor. She took me back to what I thought would be an office but instead was just a simple room which I later found out she just rented out to provide her service to clients. Gina's initial appointment was a full hour like all her appointments so thankfully I filled my paperwork out ahead of time as we probably spent ten or fifteen minutes going over it and then she used the rest of the time to give me my first treatment. When the session ended I went ahead and made my next appointment figuring if I felt a difference I would keep it. As it turned out I did continue seeing Gina and instead of relying on Dad to get me to my appointments all the time I started taking TARC. During my sessions with Gina, I quickly learned that she would talk about anything and quickly I learned that maybe she could help me sort things out in my mind about Sammi. By this time Sammi had stormed out of my exam room two or three times and played his "I don't know" game more times than I could count, and I needed to get someone else's advice. Gary could provide his input, but he was how many miles away?

By the end of 2016, I began to get the feeling, not that I had not before, that Sammi was just money hungry and while he did not get the money directly it helped the business. I thought about all the things that I saw on a regular basis when I went to the office and how he was overly demanding that I come back in this many days or weeks. Slowly I began to connect dots in regards to things I saw at the chiropractor regarding Sammi and slowly more and more things began to make sense. Then my second appointment in 2017 came around. While I had been in for one appointment in January where Sammi adjusted me three times I decided that it was time to put all the information I received in the past behind me and give Sammi a fair chance. Sammi walked into the room a few seconds after that and greeted me as usual. Having given me his email address earlier in my treatment as things were changing in my body that would not normally change with an Atlas adjustment Sammi told me to email him after my January appointment to let him know what changed. When I emailed him, on Saturday, I told him nothing changed but after being on my feet at work the following day multiple things changed, or so I thought, so I emailed him again. While I felt like I was doing the right thing Sammi asked me if I did not think those things were sufficient enough to tell him about in the first email. Having caught me off guard and sensing that he was in a bad mood about something I did not say anything. He continued making comments and at some point asked me if I was ever going to hold an adjustment again. This question totally flabbergasted me and again I did not comment. Thankfully he wound up not adjusting me, told me to make an appointment in two weeks and left the room.

When I walked up to the front desk my Mother who brought me for my appointment got up thinking she needed to pay, but since I was not adjusted did not have to. I did not say anything about what happened with Sammi, and out of instinct I just made my appointment for two weeks. After I was given my appointment card we turned to leave and I started thinking over the events of my appointment. Once in the car, though I told myself that I would just think about these things more at home and over the weekend. I figured I already made an appointment for two weeks so I told myself that I would keep it and if I did not feel like I needed it I would just call and cancel. I was already intent on changing Chiropractors as I did not feel that Sammi's comments were offensive but instead inappropriate. My parents continually told me that I would not be able to do this but I figured I would deal with that when the time came. Soon enough my two-week appointment was only a few days away however I had no neck pain so I canceled and told the receptionist that I would call back to reschedule. Then a million questions went through my mind. When I told my Dad, later that afternoon I canceled my appointment for Thursday all he said was okay. It was not until Thursday morning that I thought again about having canceled my appointment for later that day.

"I really did it," I thought, "I really am free from Sammi." "But what if," I thought again, "they will not let me change chiropractors when I am ready to reschedule?" I quickly pushed that thought out of my mind as I knew many patients there saw all three chiropractors; now that I was free I just needed some time to heal myself before returning.

In the end, I wound up taking a month off from the chiropractor and during that time I have to say my body felt many things. There were nights when I would wake up with my neck burning hot, nights when I would wake with my neck in pain (the pain was always gone by morning,) and times when my neck just felt clammy. I began feeling pain in other areas of my body too. I noticed that areas of my body often radiated heat and while I noticed this before leaving Sammi, it now seemed more pronounced. I knew that my body was healing and subconsciously I knew that what I did at the beginning of February was ultimately what was going to save me. I thought about how early on Sammi said that over adjustment can cause nerve damage and that is when the erratic patterns really began. I began thinking back to the phrase my college history professor used to quote from Lord Acton "all power corrupts and absolute power corrupts absolutely." I had fallen victim so many times in my life to this but this time I got to pick up the pieces too. In the past when things like this happened I was able to just move on, but this time I already knew that it would take time to make myself stronger. I felt things in my body on a regular basis and fortunately, I now had Gina and Gary to help me make sense of all this. While I blamed no one, I knew I still had a long way to go.

# CHAPTER FOUR

WHEN I CALLED TO RESCHEDULE MY CHIropractic appointment thankfully Sammi's sister, Beth Daken, answered the phone. Beth had taken an interest in me since the first time she met me at the office and after I said the words "I need to make an appointment with," I paused knowing that this could be a sink or swim scenario, "Toby." After I said my last word there was a pause before an answer came and all the visions I had of being able to and not being able to see a different chiropractor flashed through my mind and when Beth did say something about me not seeing Sammi to bring me back to reality I was able to come back with a response that made it appear as if I was not avoiding Sammi but simply doing what was more convenient for myself. Since my Dad had just started a new job I simply said: "it works better for my schedule."

After all, what had Sammi done to me? He did make some comments that I felt were inappropriate but nothing to make a scene about. "When did you want to come in," Beth asked.

Knowing that Toby worked Saturdays I just picked a Saturday several weeks out and when Beth said "how about 9:20 am," I said, "I will take that." Hanging up the phone I thought that was easy enough. I was able to make the change I wanted, I did not get anyone in trouble and my appointment is early enough in the morning I still have the rest of the day to do things. When Dad came home that afternoon I told him that I had an appointment with Toby on March 4th at 9:20 in the morning. He said okay but nothing more as he knew I was getting frustrated with Sammi and even though he did not know the whole story I did not feel like he needed to. When March 4th came I went in for my appointment and Toby greeted me in his style much like Sammi had done and right away I answered back with the line "you are going to adjust me." By this time I had grown accustom to using this phrase when I saw the Atlas Orthogonist as Sammi had put enough fear in me to last what felt like a lifetime not to mention confusing me in the process. Of course, this time I felt like I did have some right to say this as I had not been adjusted in over a month and undoing what was already done was not going to happen overnight. Toby wound up adjusting me twice before using the impulse gun, but he did not tell me when I had to come back. After Dad paid and I made my next appointment we walked out. On the way home I talked to Dad some about my appointment then I was silent. Toby's style was so much different from Sammi's; just right now I still had so much fear in me that I treated Toby the same way I learned to treat Sammi. When my next appointment came with Toby again I said "you are going to adjust me," and again I was adjusted two times. Then on the way home, I began thinking, "I do get benefit from being adjusted but a lot of times those benefits are only temporary, I get more benefit from seeing Gina.

Still, I was determined that I would quit neither as a little voice inside me kept telling me that both things would result in the answer for Atlas alignment. Plus I still had one thorn in my side with Dr. Von Roenn who Sammi recommended me to see for treatment with the DNA appliance while I was seeing him as a patient, and by this time I was not sure which one frustrated me more. This is where Gina came in; she not only aided in my treatment but having some dental knowledge she could provide me with insight that the regular orthodontist would not see. Gina helped me to make sense of things that for various reasons the mainstream did not want to explain and in some ways, she helped to boost my confidence and make me feel like I was not crazy. Up till now, so many people had not given me room to think and while looking at all areas of the alternative allowed me some discernment real truth came from research. Still so often I found that people tried to shut me down because of my research I learned quickly who I could talk to about what and this is when I began to feel like I was living multiple lives.

Soon enough my third appointment with Toby came and by now I was finally starting to develop the feeling that my Atlas continually going out of alignment was not my fault and actually starting to realize that Toby did not care if he had to adjust me every time or not, and I was starting to figure out that all the benefits I told Sammi I was getting were not all that lasting and it was almost as if Sammi wanted an instantaneous email update to boost his ego to make him feel like he was reinventing something that had been lying dormant for years. A few moments later Toby walked in and having made the decision to abandon my "you are going to adjust me" phrase I just greeted him. This time I figured I would just start talking natural and let things go from there. In the end, Toby did adjust me two times before using the impulse gun but this time I did not feel like it was my fault and things did seem to go a lot smoother too. On the way home I started looking at everything that my body gained but then realized for the first time that most of those gains would be lost by mid-week the following week. More proof, I thought, that Atlas adjustments were great for the short-term but were by no means the only thing I needed. The following Saturday I was back again to see Toby as I had made the decision to make an appointment with Gary the following week and wanted to be feeling my best for that. When Toby walked in he acted surprised to see me but I remained calm as I saw that he took a different approach to things and just started a conversation as usual. I explained the events of last week and why I wanted to get checked out. Toby did adjust me and by the following week when I saw Gary I had a great deal of pain in both of my legs. I do not know if that last adjustment activated my nerve pain as I had some pain before while being adjusted by Sammi but just ignored it and went on with my life. Still, that pain which I had not experienced in some time was what I thought the traditional medical spectrum would just diagnose as nerve pain or neuropathy and treat accordingly.

On the day of my appointment, my Dad and I drove into the parking lot of the hotel where Gary and Renee were staying. We passed a man sitting outside who my Dad recognized to be Gary and it looked like he was with another patient going over their scan. We parked and then went inside to sit in the lobby. Closer to my appointment time I called Renee to find out if Gary would come to get me and she said that she was out running some errands and that Gary was sitting outside by the pool with the patient before me going over their scan and he would see me when he walked by and she would be there shortly. When Gary did come through the front door I stood up and after greeting me my Dad and I followed him and once we were in front of the door to their hotel room I mentioned to Gary about the pain in my legs figuring since he was a Naturopath I should at least acknowledge it. At the time Gary did not say anything but I somehow sensed that he would take care of it. Once we were inside Gary started talking to me and a few moments later Renee appeared at the door with several bags of groceries. I stood up to hold the door while Gary continued to talk. After Renee was inside Gary stood up and there was some movement and reorganization of things. By this time Gary finished talking to me and I used that time to quickly scan the room I was sitting in. Gary's computer was hooked up to the television for his scan, Renee's computer was conveniently by their wireless printer in the corner of the room, and I noticed a mat laying on the floor and wondered if that was the Bemer mat Gary and I had talked about via email.

By this time Gary sat back down and had me sit next to him on the sofa, so I could put my hands and feet on the glass plates for the scan. Today though, for some reason, the scan was not reading me and after a few tries Gary said that was alright as he said the biofeedback scan would provide the same information. We talked for a few more minutes and then he had me lay down on the mat in the corner which as I suspected was their Bemer mat. Renee explained how to use the mat and then set the timer for 16 minutes. As I laid there Gary, Renee and I talked about various things within the Naturopathic and allopathic fields. After my time was up and I put my socks and shoes back on Renee started the biofeedback scan and once that scan was complete the report was finalized on the computer and then printed. Once the report printed Gary picked that up along with a cellular restoration page and we proceeded to head outside to go over the report. Gary began going over the report and while he did not have to go into as much detail about things, as he knew from working with me in the past and corresponding with me via email that I knew what he was talking about, he still looked at everything the report said. By this time Gary also knew that I did my own research before I did anything that he recommended that way I could choose the best course of action for me. After Gary finished going over the report he began filling out the cellular restoration page as to what products he saw best to help restore and repair my cells. He made the suggestion too that I look into purchasing a Bemer mat. While I laid on their Bemer mat inside the hotel room for the pain in my legs I actually had not thought any more about my pain and just figured that would be something I would think about once we were home. After writing Bemer mat on the cellular restoration page Gary asked if I had any other questions and I did have a few. I asked the basic questions I had fairly quickly except for the last two. I swallowed hard and asked if I was vaccine injured to which he said yes, but not having enough knowledge at the time just left it at that. The final question I stalled for what seemed like forever as I knew the answer meant a change on my part but as far as I was concerned I knew I needed the answer. "What would it take," I said after several moments, "to do what you do?"

I paused and waited for an answer pretty sure that Gary knew from reading all my emails and the way I ordered products that this was coming. While Gary tried not to smile I could tell that he was happy that someone wanted to be the type of Naturopath that he was. He told me that he studied and taught himself then went to Washington to take the test. I did not ask anything else right then and when Gary asked if I had any other questions I said that I did not. There was a pause almost as if Gary was looking for something to say himself or more so the courage to do so. Then he began telling me about the RV they bought to travel the country in and how they had gone into debt to buy that and then he started talking about diet and while I cannot remember his exact words I do remember him hinting towards the fact that you did not always have to do things one hundred percent healthy to have a healthy lifestyle. He paused again almost as if he was looking to me for help but not wanting to come directly out and say it. Then he talked to me about how two men in black came to visit him at his house and warned him to stop doing what he was doing, and while this statement sparked my interest I did not know what I could do.

After a brief pause, I paid Gary and we said our goodbyes and parted ways. Getting in the van to leave my Dad and I decided that we would drive up to a nearby Wal-Mart to get some juice for the night and maybe something small to eat as it was almost eight o'clock at night and neither one of us wanted a big meal. Being that I had a scan before there was really nothing for Dad and I to talk about regarding the scan and I was just glad that throughout the whole process he let me do my own thing and when Gary did go over the scan with me he did not involve himself in any way. Right now I just had a lot to think about and I really would not start on that until we were back home in Louisville, Kentucky.

By this time we were at Wal-Mart and we both got out of the van. My Dad walked over to get a shopping cart while I waited by the van. Once we were inside Wal-Mart we walked to find the juice aisle and picked out two small bottles of juice. We started walking towards the registers and figured if we saw anything small to eat on the way we would buy that too. We did find some ready-cooked chicken wings in the main aisle so we decided to get those that way we would have some kind of food that night. Dad paid for our items then we left. Once we were back at the hotel for the night we sat down, ate the chicken wings and drank some juice. Dad turned on the television and we talked some but not really about the scan. I was glad though as I had a lot to think about. After everything Gary talked to me about and that thinking was something I wanted to do alone and I actually probably would not start until next week. We finished the chicken and wound up drinking a whole bottle of juice, sat and talked for a few minutes then I went to get ready for bed. My Dad followed right behind me as we would be getting up early tomorrow to head back home. Morning came and Dad woke me up when he went to take a shower and I got dressed. After he dressed he started loading the van and once everything was inside we left. Sometime closer to eight o'clock we stopped at Starbucks to use the restroom, he got a coffee and I got a latte then we headed on our way. In my spare time, I thought about things but unlike the first time I knew things were going to be easier as I already had a lot of the restoration process going, and a lot of what Gary talked about regarding the scan just involved making changes and adding or subtracting things.

My final question is what would involve more research and soul searching.

We arrived home mid-afternoon and Mom was still at work but our dog Shelby was waiting for us. I let her outside and Dad unloaded the van. When Mom came home that evening she asked about our trip and Dad pretty much told her. I did insert a few details but mostly kept my thoughts to myself. I already knew she did not care about my scan and I figured next week when Dad started back to work I would start looking at things on my own as it was already mid-week and Dad and I still had plenty of things to take care of before the weekend came and he went back to work on Monday. Soon enough the new week came and once both of my parents left for the day I began looking at the restoration products that Gary recommended. I first began by comparing my previous restoration page to the new restoration page to see how Gary's recommendations changed. Already knowing what the previous restoration products did, I decided what products I wanted to keep using and what ones I no longer needed. Next, I began looking at Gary's new recommendations. I researched each product and decided what areas I wanted to focus on. By the end of the day, I compiled a list of all products old and new that I wanted to use. Products from the first scan I already had and could continue using and the new products I would order and start taking them when they arrived. The next day I began thinking about the last question I asked Gary. As of right now I knew I had nowhere to start but I needed to collect my thoughts before I emailed Gary.

Once I collected my thoughts I emailed Gary. I sent him the website I told him I would and asked one other question that came into my mind since my appointment. I asked him if he would go ahead and send me the information he had on the Bemer mat as I probably would end up getting one after I did my own research and then I asked if he could send me some of the titles of the books he used to get where he is today. As I clicked the send button I realized there was no turning back now just self-teaching. I had taken an online course in college and liked it very much but there you still had an instructor that put up notes, gave assignments with deadlines and told you what to study. Here I would have the material, have to figure out what I need to know and set my own dates, not to mention still trying to improve my own health and look into the vaccine injury question. I went to bed that night thinking all these things and for the first time feeling a little bit overwhelmed; still, I woke the next morning with a clearer mind and the thought that once I had titles of books I could move forward as I chose. I spent that day and the rest of the week gathering my thoughts about my life and adding things to my personal To-Do list that I needed to get done that I had been stalling on forever. Still after having everything, so to speak, thrown in my face back in February 2017 my eyes were opened to a lot of things and I realized how much had been kept from me all my life. I continued writing things on my

To-Do list and figured when Gary answered me back I would go online and buy the books he recommended and once my life was together I would start studying. Friday came and I saw Gina. I told her about my appointment with Gary and how what showed up were sharp sticky pains primarily in my lower legs pushing my hip up thus causing my Atlas to go out of alignment, or at least make it seem that way. Making this statement to Gina was the first time I realized that what I thought all along was right and every time Sammi adjusted me my Atlas may not have been out of alignment.

# CHAPTER FIVE

SATURDAY I SAW TOBY AND HE ADJUSTED my Atlas as coming back from my scan everything was still too new and while it had been almost two weeks since my scan after the revelation I had when I talked to Gina it seemed like the tables were turning. I talked to Toby as usual and even told him that Gary agreed that I was vaccine injured and even though I was happy to know this information Toby seemed surprised that I was glad I was vaccine injured. I was not so much glad to know this information but, as I told Toby, at least I had a place to start. Toby asked me if my parents knew and I said no. He did not ask if I was going to tell them, but now that question entered my mind. After that conversation, a few more things were said then I went to checkout. For the first time going home, I realized that aside from my body feeling better I gained nothing from the adjustment even though when I arrived home I would try to convince myself I did. This thought started me thinking, other than the first few times, when I truly was in pain, I really did not gain anything from being adjusted by Sammi other than like he said early on nerve damage. When we arrived home I started on things I wanted to do that day and left thoughts about the chiropractor for the following week. Toby did not go overboard adjusting me and while the first two times involved two Atlas adjustments we were now down to one and the way I looked at it is the first time I probably needed two adjustments. When the new week came around I saw that Gary emailed me back so I took care of that email first. Once that was out of the way I began thinking about the chiropractor and honestly in some ways, thanks to Sammi, this thought was bigger than me. The more I thought about it the more upset I became as I realized that Sammi knew what he was doing. He might not have known in the beginning but after he started making progress something had to kick in. While this thought plagued me for the rest of the week soon enough I went to see Gina. As it had been for several months now Gina was my sounding board, helping me to make sense of this whole thing and during my appointments with Sammi I quickly learned to just tell him what he wanted and at this point, I still treated Toby that way.

    My next appointment was my last appointment with Toby for the year and again he adjusted my Atlas. By now I told him that I really did not get benefit out being adjusted and he probably more or less did it to pacify me. When I went in for my first appointment in the New Year Toby made the comment that my right leg was ¼ of an inch short. He noted that it had been this way all along when he adjusted me to make my legs even. He asked me how I was feeling and when I told him that I was feeling fine he asked if I wanted him to adjust me. I paused not knowing what to say. With Sammi, I hardly ever got out of an adjustment and if I did it was for a reason that Sammi could explain. Toby went on to explain that whenever he adjusted me I always came back with my right leg ¼ of an inch short. While at the time I did not understand it I told him not to adjust me and I figured we would see what happened. Toby went on to tell me about another patient he had whose legs were not even but whose body was happy and that is when it clicked for me that for right now this might be where my body needs to be, with one leg a little longer than the other, and if my body does become even it will do so on its own or with the help of Craniosacral therapy. After Toby finished talking to me I went to checkout as today I only needed to make my next appointment as I did not owe anything since I was not adjusted. "When do you want to come back," Samatha asked, and I paused for a moment not having thought about this ahead of time and I quickly thought. I normally had been scheduling appointments every seven weeks, but given that I was not adjusted today I really did not want to wait seven weeks and seven was not an even number to divide so after a moment I quickly responded four. I figured this way my body would have four weeks to adjust to no Atlas adjustment, and if not getting adjusted was not the right thing for my body I would not have to wait a full seven weeks before coming back in.

When I saw Gina at the end of the month I told her what Toby did at my last appointment and while she did seem a bit surprised she just went about how she reviewed things for her appointment. I was not alarmed by this as I knew by now Gina took an interest in my chiropractic care she just had her own job to do, and like me knew that in due time things would work themselves out. Gina noted as she had on several other occasions that my left hip was higher than my right and I told her how my body felt, but I did admit that my body did feel better not having had my Atlas adjusted.

The following Saturday I saw Toby and when he walked in the room the first thing he asked was how I did after not being adjusted last time. I told him that my body did not feel as tense and it seemed easier to do things. After this Toby checked my legs as well as my neck and having talked to me during previous visits about other things asked me if I wanted him to adjust me this time just to see what happens. I thought for a few moments about the body from a Naturopathic standpoint and came to the decision that I would let Toby adjust me based on knowing that the adjustment would eventually wear off and my body would bounce back if there was a negative impact. After Toby adjusted me as well as using the impulse gun we talked for a few minutes and then I went to checkout. After my Dad paid for today's adjustment Samatha asked me when I wanted to come back in and having thought the whole thing out while I was waiting to make sure the adjustment held I calmly responded five weeks. I figured that was enough time to tell if the adjustment was good or bad for my body. By the next morning paying more attention to the results from the adjustment I noticed that all the immediate results were starting to disappear and I had a sense of tension beginning to build in my body. This tension in my body increased as the first week went on and by the end of the week, everything gained from the adjustment was gone. When I saw Gina the following week I told her what Toby and I agreed upon. I did not tell her about the tension I had in my whole body but instead just my chief complaints and I learned later that the tension played directly into my complaints. I saw Gina two more times before this final statement finally began making sense for me, and that is when I realized that having my Atlas continually adjusted was hindering me more than helping me; and prior to changing chiropractors, was even having a detrimental effect on my body. I, for the first time, saw all the negative effects continual Atlas adjustments had on my body and while I had thought this before and even did some research into it I did not give it the attention I should have until now.

When I saw Toby, two days after Gina, he asked what the adjustment had done for me and I told him. Thinking things through in my mind as I talked I realized that no good really came out of being adjusted other than the initial relief of pain and whatever was gained was almost as quickly lost leaving my body to deal with whatever aftereffects came from it. All the negative effects, as I told Toby, began to subside at the beginning of this week like I thought they would and while Toby began talking after this I continued thinking in my mind "coming every two weeks and being adjusted barely allowed for the numbness to wear off." Now all the pieces were starting to fall into place allowing things to make sense. Toby checked my legs to find my right leg a quarter of an inch short like always. Then Toby checked my neck and when nothing was sore or tender to me when he palpated either side he began to talk to me again and what he said actually made sense. After we agreed that this might be where my body needs to be Toby asked me if anything was bothering me. While I found this to be a little weird it seemed to make more sense than whatever Sammi was doing. Toby wound up using the impulse gun on my upper and mid-back then sent me on my way. After I made my next appointment we left and I started thinking, "this concept actually makes sense. If the body is happy then why change it. Whatever happened to good old fashioned talk therapy anyway?" Still, I knew that this whole concept would take some getting used to.

# CHAPTER SIX

ONCE I WAS HOME I LOOKED AT MY APpointment card again in disbelief as I could not believe that I scheduled ten weeks out. Up till now, I had gone four and at most seven but never ten. I was slowly getting used to having control of my chiropractic care instead of having the chiropractor dictate what I did and what I needed. For the first time, I told myself "if I need to see Toby sooner I will just make an appointment. If it turns out that appointment is during the week I will go. After all, it is about me, my health and wellbeing." This is when I realized all the fear that Sammi put in me. I kept myself from doing things for fear that it might make my Atlas go out of alignment giving way for another adjustment(s) upon my next visit. After ten weeks I quickly allowed myself to graduate to twelve weeks just to see what would happen. I still maintained my quarter of an inch difference thus determining that this is where my body wanted to stay for now. After this, I went back to scheduling appointments ten weeks apart figuring that now that my body had time to overcome things, namely fear, everything else would come together in due time. In the meantime, I would see Gina every two weeks and Toby every ten weeks just to get checked.

My conversations with Toby gradually became easier after he stopped my continual adjustments and I figured out that I could talk about Naturopathic matters with him too. We agreed upon the idea that a quarter of an inch off was where my body needed to be right now and, I added, if any other changes happened they would happen on their own or with the help of Craniosacral therapy. While I did not fully understand my last statement and Toby did not comment I knew that craniosacral therapy was the answer; after all why else would Sammi have gotten so upset and defensive about me trying a different approach?

From here on out my legs remained a quarter of an inch different but my body was happy and guess what ultimately Toby was happy. At my appointments, Toby always asked me if there was anything bothering me and if so he normally focused on that area with the impulse gun. If nothing was bothering me, Toby, normally just used the impulse gun to adjust my spine as well as the rest of my back. On several occasions towards the end of 2018, Gina noted how level my hips were given all the time and effort I put in. At the time I did not think anything about this statement other than to say "my body is healing."

It was not until I saw Toby for the first time in 2019 and he made the comment that my hips and pelvis are the straightest that they have ever been since he started seeing me in March of 2017 that it really sank in. "My body is really healing," I thought, "and things that were done are being undone." By this time Toby asked me to "please sit" so he could palpate my neck to see if anything was sore there and that is when I figured I would think more about this comment later right now I just carried on a conversation with Toby and once he was done I went to checkout, made my appointment for ten weeks and left with my Dad. I talked to him the way home and figured once I was home and upstairs I would have plenty of time to think while I worked on other things. I realized, as I had told myself many times, things were falling into place and while I had been collecting bits and pieces of information all along soon I would have the final remaining pieces of the puzzle to confirm what I envisioned for quite some time.

The next time I saw Gina I told her what Toby said at my appointment and while she was not surprised I could tell that she was glad for me. "All my hard work is finally paying off," I thought, "and if Sammi was just willing to work with me…." I paused and quickly snapped myself back into reality "this is not what I am here for and I can think about these matters later." I began telling Gina my complaints and I mentioned the number of times I had fallen over the past two weeks. Of course, I made sure to mention what I noticed after the last time I fell. From here I began noticing things seemed to change at a more accelerated pace and every change seemed to be a change for the better. Shortly into the month of April, I noticed that I was starting to sleep better for the first time in years, probably since before my aneurysm, and I made sure to mention this. While talking I realized this is probably why I was miserable in my life up till now as I was significantly lacking quality sleep in my life. The day before Easter I told Gina that I had fallen again this time hitting the middle of the base of the back of my skull on the side of a wooden table. While I hit fairly hard and wound up sitting down with my legs crossed in a not so pretty fashion the first sensation I felt was an instantaneous sensation of pain then I paused in my mind and asked myself what just happened. A little voice inside me said, "something good just happened." Again I paused this time as if drawing a large question mark in my mind all the while asking myself what I could have gained. The base of my skull was now incredibly sore but things felt different primarily in my neck. Gina noted that I had a noticeable knot on my head where I hit which thankfully my hair covered up; still, she worked on helping to heal the area. During the session, I noted that this last fall changed something significant, and hopefully, when I saw Toby on Saturday I would find out some "good news". Soon enough Saturday came and treating it just like any other Saturday I did my usual in the morning. My Dad and I left for the chiropractor the same time as always and I put any thought I had about something good happening out of my mind allowing myself to focus on the here and now. When we arrived at the chiropractor I signed in and Samantha sent me back to an exam room right away and on the way back I was greeted by Toby who followed me into the room. He asked me the usual questions and then had me lay down so he could check my legs and that was when, after a few moments, I asked if my right leg was still ¼ of an inch short. He continued moving my legs around and said nothing at first then after an extended pause told me that my right leg was now 1/8 of an inch short. When I heard these words for the first time it shocked me, but then I realized all the hard work I was doing and the pain that I tolerated was worth it and things, as I told myself in the beginning, were finding ways to fix themselves.

Toby finished the exam and after I checked out I told my Dad the news, while we were driving home, from the appointment today. While I was happy with the news he did not seem that impressed, other than to make a few comments. Still, I was happy and nothing was going to get me down. Once we were home I went to start doing what I needed to do that day and did not think much more about my appointment other than to make a few notes. "My body was healing on its own," I thought, "and while it had been doing so for a while it is nice to know that my legs were finally becoming even." Now came the time when many new questions began to enter my mind about things my body felt and experienced before that I just brushed off or made up some logical explanation for as I was too busy dealing with other issues or putting up with "I don't know" man to actually research or talk to my Naturopath about, and since it was already late in 2018 and I knew that I wanted to try to get another scan next year I would wait to see if that appointment would come to be before I started asking my questions via email.

# CHAPTER SEVEN

THE REMAINING MONTHS OF 2018 SEEMED to pass by quickly and the first few months of 2019 turned out to do the same. While I emailed Gary back in mid-December of 2018 about the possibility of another scan sometime next year the answer I received then was no and I figured I would just wait and see what God had in store. By now I had the first three books that Gary recommended, which I later determined were the foundation for studying Naturopathic medicine, still I had not even opened one so maybe the answer of no was some sort of sign that I already had all the answers and just needed a force greater than myself to guide me. With that said good news came from Renee in March of 2019. Gary received a new scanner to replace the old one whose license expired around this time last year. Reading this news I thought "this is why Gary said no back in December," and while my mind wandered back to our conversation back in 2017 I told myself "just go ahead and try to set up a scan." I contacted Renee the following day and she told me their current plans. She asked me where I lived and I told her. After almost being hung up on because I did not live anywhere near the areas they were going to do scans I did manage to get out the phrase "we are willing to drive." Back in 2012 I came to the realization the allopathic realm was not going to heal or cure me and right now the type of care I needed either had to be done long distance or with travel. Still there was a brief pause on the other end of the phone before Renee began telling me places they were going to around Kentucky.

Renee said they were stopping in Pennsylvania then heading to New York and either coming back to Pennsylvania or going to Baltimore. The first dates that they were going to be in Pennsylvania were too short of notice for us to get there. New York was even a further drive so that was out of the question. With that said I told Renee to let me know if they were coming back to Pennsylvania or going to Baltimore and left it at that. Dad said if nothing came of either of those he would take me to Wilmington, North Carolina which was going to be their last stop. As it turned out after New York they went back to Pennsylvania for an even shorter time then headed back to Florida before heading to Wilmington. Gary passed away shortly after they returned to Florida.

Renee's mother was the one that sent out the letter that Renee wrote to alert all Gary's patients of the news and upon reading the letter the morning of the first Tuesday in July I have to say that I was not overly alarmed by the news and started thinking what I needed to do. Whether it was because of the restoration products I was using since 2017 or something else I, for the first time, did not feel like I had to jump into panic mode. I knew I wanted to print the letter for my Dad to read as he had taken me both times I saw Gary and he would not go jumping to conclusions and I wanted to send a message to the host of the Internet program, Vinnie Johanson, I listen to in order to let him know that Gary died; the rest could wait until tomorrow. Once I finished reviewing my email I went back to print Renee's letter and after that, I took a break from things and when I resumed what I was doing I began typing my message to Vinnie. In my message I included the letter Renee wrote and once I was satisfied I clicked send. Then I shut my laptop down and went downstairs to take care of things that I needed to. Other than leaving the printed letter for my Dad to read I really did not think anymore about Gary other than to answer questions for my Dad when he read the letter from Renee as I had not told him everything about Gary before my visit with him in 2015, but I really did not feel like I needed to.

The next day when I started looking at things I looked at the letter Renee sent out about Gary's death. In the letter, she described how and where Gary died. Then I opened the letter I saved from Renee in March and reviewed that, and then I thought back to the conversation Gary and I had back in 2017 after reviewing my scan. While my first question "Am I vaccine-injured?" was a question that I needed to know the answer to; weight sat on my second question and events in Gary's life primarily from 2015 till now. "How do I do what you do?" was the question that my mind rested on for some time before I again looked at the letter regarding Gary's death. At this point the picture became clearer as to why Gary's face lit up and his smile grew immensely during our conversation in 2017. During our talk Gary noted that two men in black came to visit him at his house telling him to stop what he was doing or else. While Renee did not mention anything about the men in black in her final statement regarding Gary I began to look at them as the precursor to all the events that followed. The men in black and their statement, his scanner, and ultimately his choice to push forward; yes it was time to move Gary out of the picture. Whether Gary's reliance on allopathic medicine came in 2015 or 2017 was beside the point but still the mainstream had to make it appear as such and now they had to begin planning things carefully to make it as if Gary died naturally. Up till now holistic individuals had been found dead anywhere but at home however with Gary's whole business about travel the thought of him dying on the road just seemed too unnatural therefore he had to die at home. Once I concluded the final statement though I thought little more about this as I knew no one in my immediate circle would believe me and while they might listen to me nothing else would come of it other than frustration on my part. I did send my thoughts to Vinnie but did little else with the information that I concluded.

Now that I had thought things through and came to my own conclusions based on the information I had I made the decision that I was going to stay doing things through a naturopathic model as I had come too far now to turn back to allopathic and mainstream ways, and like I told Gina I probably would just have to suck it up for a while. I learned a lot from Gary both in person as well as over the Internet and, at this point, I felt like I could pick up whatever information I lacked in a new Naturopath. With this said I told Gina what happened and asked her if she knew of any Naturopathic doctors and at the end of the session she gave me the name of a health practitioner as well as a Naturopathic doctor. Doing research over the next few days I came to quickly realize that if I wanted to continue making progress I needed the Naturopathic doctor and I would just have to willingly start teaching myself just like Gary did.

# CHAPTER EIGHT

I CONTACTED THE NATUROPATHIC DOCTOR who Gina referred me to as I just wanted to ask a couple of questions however she was ready to set up a new patient appointment. Not thinking things through I went ahead and gave her my phone number so that she could call me to set up an appointment. It was not until I spoke with Denise the first time that I realized I was rushing into things. While I did not make an appointment with Denise on the phone, the following day I emailed her and told her to put my appointment on hold. Gina had given me her name less than two weeks ago, Gary had not been out of the picture even a month yet and as far as I was concerned I just had a lot on my plate right now and needed to make some choices before worrying about a new Naturopath. I still had things I wanted to sort through in my mind and things I needed to take care of before I worried about another new appointment. I stayed busy for the remainder of July and the beginning portion of August before deciding to contact Denise again. Of course it did not help matters any that Renee called me the last full week of July explaining that they were in Wilmington doing scans. At that moment a million questions came into my mind and while I started asking them I could tell that Renee's temper was running short so I just finished things up with my story from 2017 and when that went over Renee's head just left things at that, said I would not be able to make it there for a scan and hung up. Again a million questions went through my mind with the biggest one being how she could keep doing what Gary did with no knowledge to base it on. I looked on the website Linkedin as I knew they both had profiles on this site. I saw the difference in profiles and again asked myself how? I still wanted to help Renee but began to realize that she was playing with Pandora's Box and one move the wrong way and something was going to happen. I talked to my Dad when he came home about my phone call from Renee and explained my thoughts with him agreeing. The next time I saw Gina I told her about the call and for the first time realized that while I wanted to help Renee I needed to find a new Naturopath. I had been caught in the middle before with Sammi and did not need to have Renee do that to me again.

With that said I turned down Renee a total of two more times before finally making the decision to contact Denise. I made a New Patient appointment for the end of September and did receive one more call from Renee before they headed off to the West Coast. During this call, I told Renee that I really could not meet her for a scan and, not directly, told her no. I knew in my mind that what Renee was doing was not right and wanted to stay out of it as much as I could. If our paths happened to cross I would worry about things then. For now I had my appointment with Denise at the end of September and I would see what came of that. Right now I had Gary's protocol to continue to follow and when my appointment came I would proceed from there. Gina already told me that Denise used Biofeedback and I figured I would talk to her about things from Gary.

When the day came for my appointment with Denise I rode TARC 3 there and really did not think about the appointment until I arrived there. The office, while it was bigger than Gina's, was only for Denise but having multiple rooms allowed for her to make the most out of her day as after the initial new patient visit which included biofeedback you came back for three additional Rife sessions which only entailed her setting the machine and then it basically took care of itself. Still, Denise, as Gary put it, was basically a one-man band running to all the rooms throughout the day and managing all the tasks that multiple employees do in a mainstream office. Again I was reminded of Gary's statement of how all Denise can do is plant seeds and hope they are picked up and built on. With that thought in my mind, as I sat with the light for the Rife machine on my lap, I knew I was doing the right thing in starting to work with Denise. I was initially giving up on curing all dis-ease but in the end knew that I would be healing my body but at a different level. Again I told myself I was doing this for me and right now I figured I would continue ordering product from the shipping department that Gary used as Denise did not have a problem with me doing that and should the need arise order those products from other websites I knew where to find them. Gary knew that I thoroughly researched any of his products before I started using them much like how I thought through my questions before asking them. With this thought in my mind I just sat back and finished the Rife session as I was now content with the fact that I as well as Gary knew what I was doing.

www.ingramcontent.com/pod-product-compliance
Lightning Source LLC
LaVergne TN
LVHW011859060526
838200LV00054B/4417